PARKINSON
DIET RECIPES
COOKBOOK

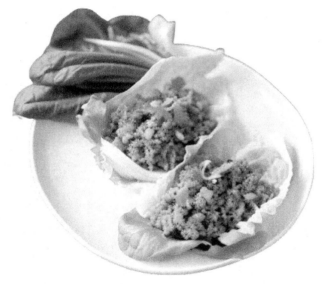

Ultimate Dietary Guide with 20 Delicious Recipes
to Manage and Reverse Parkinson's Disease for
Newly Diagnosed

Dixie McCoy

Copyright © 2023 by Dixie McCoy

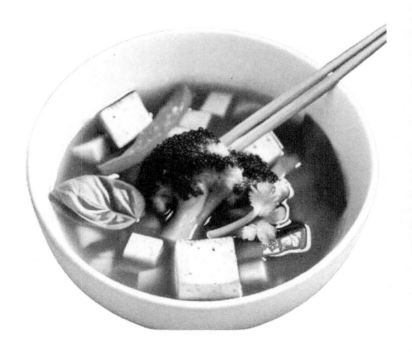

TABLE OF CONTENT

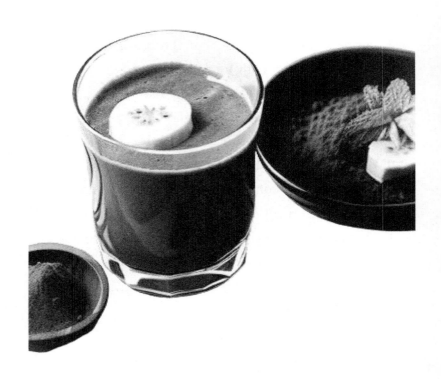

Introduction

Meet John, a 40-year-old man who had been diagnosed with early-onset Parkinson's disease. He was devastated when he found out and was determined to find a way to manage his symptoms without relying solely on medication.

After months of research, John stumbled upon an unusual approach—a diet that consisted primarily of fermented foods. The theory behind this diet was that the probiotics in fermented foods could improve gut health, which in turn could reduce inflammation and improve brain function.

John was skeptical but decided to give it a try. He started incorporating fermented foods like kefir, kimchi, and sauerkraut into his diet. To his surprise, he noticed a significant improvement in his symptoms. His tremors reduced, his mood improved, and he felt more energized.

John's neurologist was intrigued by his progress and started researching the link between gut health and Parkinson's disease. He discovered that there is evidence to suggest that the gut-brain connection plays a significant role in the development and progression of Parkinson's disease.

John now swears by his fermented food diet and has become an advocate for using alternative approaches to manage Parkinson's disease. He even started a blog to share his experience and help others who are struggling with the disease.

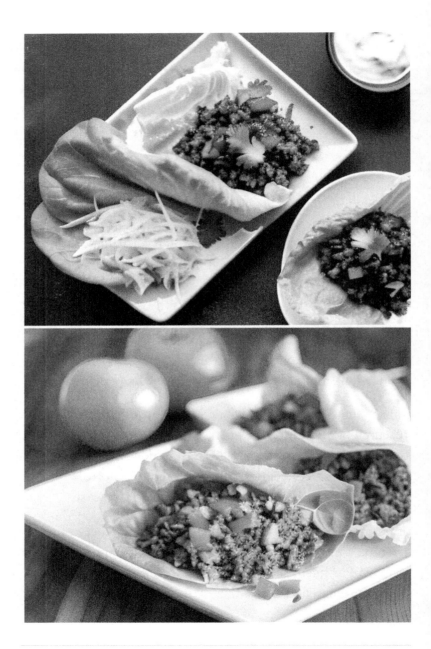

DELICIOUS ANTI-PARKINSON DIET RECIPES

1. Fermented Kefir Smoothie Bowl

Prep Time: 5 minutes

Ingredients:

- 1 cup kefir
- 1 frozen banana
- 1/2 cup mixed berries
- 1 tablespoon chia seeds
- 1 tablespoon honey (optional)
- Toppings: sliced fruits, nuts, and granola

Instructions:

1. In a blender, combine kefir, frozen banana, mixed berries, chia seeds, and honey (if using).
2. Blend until smooth and creamy.
3. Pour the smoothie into a bowl.
4. Top with sliced fruits, nuts, and granola.
5. Enjoy the fermented kefir smoothie bowl immediately.

2. Kimchi Fried Rice

Prep Time: 15 minutes

Ingredients:

- 2 cups cooked rice (preferably day-old)
- 1 cup kimchi, chopped
- 1/2 cup cooked protein (such as chicken, shrimp, or tofu), diced

- 2 tablespoons vegetable oil
- 2 cloves garlic, minced
- 1/2 cup frozen mixed vegetables
- 2 tablespoons soy sauce
- 1 tablespoon sesame oil
- 2 green onions, chopped
- Salt and pepper to taste

Instructions:

1. Use a large skillet or wok to heat vegetable oil on medium heat setting.

2. Add finely chopped garlic and cook over medium heat for approximately 60 seconds or until it releases its pleasant aroma.

3. Add chopped kimchi and cooked protein. Stir-fry for 2-3 minutes.

4. Add frozen mixed vegetables and continue stir-frying for another 2 minutes.

5. Add cooked rice to the skillet and break up any clumps with a spatula.

6. Gradually pour soy sauce and sesame oil over the rice, ensuring a well-distributed coating. Stir well to combine.

7. Cook for an additional 3-4 minutes until the rice is heated through.

8. Enhance the flavor by adding salt and pepper to your liking.

9. Remove from heat and garnish with chopped green onions.

10. Serve the kimchi fried rice hot.

3. Sauerkraut and Turkey Lettuce Wraps

Prep Time: 10 minutes

Ingredients:

- 8 large lettuce leaves (such as iceberg or romaine)
- 1 cup sauerkraut
- 1/2 pound ground turkey
- 1 tablespoon olive oil
- 1/2 onion, finely chopped
- 2 cloves garlic, minced
- 1/2 teaspoon ground cumin
- 1/2 teaspoon paprika
- Salt and pepper to taste
- Optional toppings: chopped tomatoes, avocado, and cilantro

Instructions:

1. Heat olive oil in a skillet over medium heat.
2. Add chopped onion and minced garlic. Cook over medium heat until aromatic and onions become see-through.
3. Add ground turkey and cook until browned, breaking it up with a spatula.
4. Stir in ground cumin, paprika, salt, and pepper.
5. Cook for an additional 2-3 minutes until the turkey is fully cooked.
6. Remove from heat and set aside.
7. Wash and dry the lettuce leaves.

8. Spoon a generous amount of sauerkraut onto each lettuce leaf.

9. Top with the cooked ground turkey mixture.

10. Add optional toppings like chopped tomatoes, avocado, and cilantro.

11. Roll up the lettuce leaves and secure with toothpicks if needed.

12. Serve the sauerkraut and turkey lettuce wraps as a refreshing appetizer or light meal.

4. Fermented Pickle and Salmon Salad

Prep Time: 10 minutes

Ingredients:

- 2 cups mixed salad greens
- 4 ounces cooked salmon, flaked
- 1/2 cup fermented pickles, sliced
- 1/4 red onion, thinly sliced
- 1/4 cup cherry tomatoes, halved
- 2 tablespoons extra virgin olive oil
- 2 tablespoons lemon juice
- Salt and pepper to taste

Instructions:

1. In a large bowl, combine the mixed salad greens, flaked salmon, sliced fermented pickles, red onion, and cherry tomatoes.

2. Combine the extra virgin olive oil and lemon juice in a small bowl, gently blending them with a whisk.

3. Delicately pour the dressing over the salad, gently tossing the mixture to ensure every component is evenly coated.

4. Enhance the flavor by adding salt and pepper to your liking.

5. Transfer the salad to a serving plate or bowl.

6. Enjoy the fermented pickle and salmon salad as a light and nutritious meal.

5. Tempeh Stir-Fry with Vegetables

Prep Time: 15 minutes

Ingredients:

- 8 ounces tempeh, cubed
- 2 tablespoons soy sauce
- 1 tablespoon sesame oil
- 1 tablespoon vegetable oil
- 2 cloves garlic, minced
- 1/2 onion, sliced
- 1 bell pepper, sliced
- 1 cup broccoli florets
- 1 carrot, sliced
- 1/2 cup snap peas
- 2 tablespoons hoisin sauce
- 1 tablespoon rice vinegar
- 1/2 teaspoon red pepper flakes (optional)
- Salt and pepper to taste
- 2 green onions, chopped (for garnish)

Instructions:
1. In a bowl, marinate the tempeh cubes in soy sauce and sesame oil for 10 minutes.
2. Use a large skillet or wok to heat vegetable oil on medium heat setting.
3. Add minced garlic and sliced onion. Sauté for 1-2 minutes until fragrant.
4. Add the marinated tempeh cubes to the skillet. Cook for a brief duration of 5 to 6 minutes until a slight browning effect is visible.
5. Add sliced bell pepper, broccoli florets, carrot slices, and snap peas to the skillet. Continue to stir-fry the vegetables for an additional 4-5 minutes until they reach a delightful state of tender-crispness.
6. In a small bowl, whisk together hoisin sauce, rice vinegar, red pepper flakes (if using), salt, and pepper.
7. Pour the sauce over the stir-fry and toss to coat the vegetables and tempeh.
8. Cook for an additional 1-2 minutes to heat the sauce.
9. Remove from heat and garnish with chopped green onions.
10. Serve the tempeh stir-fry with vegetables over cooked rice or noodles.

6. Miso Soup with Tofu and Vegetables

Prep Time: 10 minutes

Ingredients:

- 4 cups vegetable broth
- 2 tablespoons miso paste
- 1 cup tofu, cubed
- 1 cup sliced mushrooms
- 1 cup sliced bok choy or spinach
- 2 green onions, chopped
- 1 tablespoon soy sauce
- 1 teaspoon sesame oil
- Optional: seaweed, for garnish

Instructions:

1. In a pot, bring the vegetable broth to a simmer over medium heat.
2. In a small bowl, dilute the miso paste with a few tablespoons of hot broth, stirring until smooth.
3. Add the diluted miso paste, tofu cubes, sliced mushrooms, and bok choy (or spinach) to the pot.
4. Cook for 5-6 minutes until the vegetables are tender and the tofu is heated through.
5. Stir in chopped green onions, soy sauce, and sesame oil.
6. Sample the flavor of the dish and make appropriate seasoning adjustments, if deemed necessary.
7. Ladle the miso soup into bowls.
8. Garnish with seaweed if desired.
9. Serve the miso soup hot as a comforting and nourishing meal.

7. Fermented Beet and Carrot Salad

Prep Time: 10 minutes

Ingredients:

- 2 medium beets, grated
- 2 medium carrots, grated
- 1/4 cup apple cider vinegar
- 2 tablespoons olive oil
- 1 tablespoon honey or maple syrup
- 1 teaspoon Dijon mustard
- Salt and pepper to taste

Instructions:

1. In a large bowl, combine the grated beets and carrots.

2. In a separate small bowl, whisk together the apple cider vinegar, olive oil, honey (or maple syrup), Dijon mustard, salt, and pepper.

3. Pour the dressing over the grated beets and carrots.

4. Toss well to evenly coat the vegetables with the dressing.

5. Allow the salad to marinate for at least 10 minutes to allow the flavors to meld.

6. Serve the fermented beet and carrot salad chilled as a refreshing side dish or as a topping for sandwiches or wraps.

8. Yogurt and Berry Parfait

Prep Time: 5 minutes

Ingredients:

- 1 cup Greek yogurt
- 1 cup of mixed berries, comprising strawberries, blueberries, and raspberries
- 2 tablespoons honey or maple syrup
- 1/4 cup granola

Instructions:

1. In a glass or a bowl, layer Greek yogurt, mixed berries, and honey (or maple syrup).
2. Continue layering the ingredients until they have all been utilized, ending in a final layer consisting of a medley of assorted berries.
3. Sprinkle granola over the top for added crunch.
4. Serve the yogurt and berry parfait immediately as a nutritious and satisfying breakfast or snack.

9. Fermented Cucumber and Avocado Sushi Rolls

Prep Time: 20 minutes

Ingredients:

- 4 nori sheets
- 2 cups cooked sushi rice
- 1/2 cucumber, sliced into thin strips
- 1 ripe avocado, sliced
- 1 tablespoon rice vinegar
- Soy sauce and wasabi, for serving

Instructions:
1. Place a nori sheet on a bamboo sushi mat or a clean kitchen towel.
2. Apply a delicate coating of prepared sushi rice onto the nori sheet, ensuring to leave a narrow margin around the edges.
3. Lay cucumber and avocado slices in a line across the center of the rice.
4. Sprinkle rice vinegar over the filling.
5. Roll the nori tightly using the sushi mat or kitchen towel, applying gentle pressure to ensure a tight roll.
6. Carry out the process again using the remaining nori sheets and ingredients
7. Slice each roll into bite-sized pieces using a sharp knife.
8. Serve the fermented cucumber and avocado sushi rolls with soy sauce and wasabi for dipping.

10. Turmeric and Ginger Fermented Carrot Soup

Prep Time: 15 minutes
Cook Time: 25 minutes
Ingredients:
- 2 tablespoons olive oil
- 1 onion, chopped
- 2 cloves garlic, minced
- 1 tablespoon grated fresh ginger
- 1 teaspoon ground turmeric
- 4 cups vegetable broth
- 4 cups grated carrots

- 1 cup coconut milk
- Salt and pepper to taste
- Chopped fresh cilantro or parsley for garnish

Instructions:
1. Use a large pot to heat olive oil on medium heat setting.
2. Add chopped onion and sauté for 5 minutes until softened.
3. Add minced garlic, grated ginger, and ground turmeric. Continue cooking for an extra 2 minutes or until it releases a delightful aroma.
4. Pour in vegetable broth and add grated carrots. Bring to a boil.
5. Lower the heat to a minimum level, place a lid on the pot, and allow the contents to gently simmer for about 20 minutes until the carrots become tender.
6. Using an immersion blender or a countertop blender, puree the soup until smooth.
7. Return the soup to the pot and stir in coconut milk.
8. Enhance the flavor by adding salt and pepper to your liking.
9. Heat the soup over low heat for a few more minutes to warm it through.
10. Ladle the turmeric and ginger fermented carrot soup into bowls.
11. Garnish with chopped fresh cilantro or parsley.
12. Serve the soup hot as a comforting and flavorful meal.

11. Fermented Black Bean Tacos with Guacamole

Prep Time: 20 minutes
Ingredients:

For the fermented black beans:
- 1 can black beans, rinsed and drained
- 2 tablespoons lime juice
- 1/2 teaspoon ground cumin
- 1/2 teaspoon chili powder
- Salt and pepper to taste

For the guacamole:
- 2 ripe avocados
- 1/4 cup diced red onion
- 1/4 cup chopped fresh cilantro
- 1 tablespoon lime juice
- Salt and pepper to taste

For the tacos:
- 8 small corn tortillas
- 1 cup shredded lettuce
- 1/2 cup diced tomatoes
- 1/4 cup diced red onion
- Optional toppings: sour cream, shredded cheese, salsa

Instructions:
1. In a bowl, mash the rinsed and drained black beans with a fork until partially mashed but still chunky.
2. Add lime juice, ground cumin, chili powder, salt, and pepper to the mashed black beans. Stir well to combine. Set aside.
3. In another bowl, mash the avocados until creamy but still slightly chunky.
4. Stir in diced red onion, chopped cilantro, lime juice, salt, and pepper. Mix well to combine. Set aside.
5. Heat a non-stick skillet over medium heat and warm the corn tortillas for about 1 minute on each side until soft and pliable.
6. To assemble the tacos, spread a spoonful of fermented black beans onto each tortilla.
7. Top with shredded lettuce, diced tomatoes, and diced red onion.
8. Spoon a generous amount of guacamole over the veggies.
9. Add optional toppings like sour cream, shredded cheese, or salsa if desired.
10. Fold the tortillas in half and serve the fermented black bean tacos immediately.

12. Fermented Quinoa Salad with Roasted Vegetables

Prep Time: 15 minutes
Cook Time: 25 minutes
Ingredients:

- 1 cup quinoa, rinsed
- 2 cups vegetable broth
- 2 cups diced mixed vegetables (such as bell peppers, zucchini, and eggplant)
- 2 tablespoons olive oil
- 1 teaspoon of dried herbs, including options like thyme, rosemary, or oregano
- Salt and pepper to taste
- 2 tablespoons lemon juice
- 2 tablespoons balsamic vinegar
- 1/4 cup crumbled feta cheese (optional)
- 2 tablespoons chopped fresh parsley

Instructions:
1. Preheat the oven to 400°F (200°C).
2. In a saucepan, combine the quinoa and vegetable broth. Bring to a boil, then reduce heat to low, cover, and simmer for 15 minutes or until the quinoa is tender and the broth is absorbed.
3. While the quinoa is cooking, spread the diced mixed vegetables on a baking sheet. Drizzle with olive oil, sprinkle with dried herbs, salt, and pepper. Toss to coat evenly.

4. The vegetables should be roasted in the preheated oven for approximately 20-25 minutes, making sure to stir them once in the middle of the cooking process, until they reach a tender and lightly caramelized state.

5. In a large bowl, combine the cooked quinoa, roasted vegetables, lemon juice, and balsamic vinegar. Toss gently to mix.

6. Season with additional salt and pepper if needed.

7. Sprinkle crumbled feta cheese (if using) and chopped fresh parsley over the salad.

8. Serve the fermented quinoa salad with roasted vegetables as a nutritious and satisfying side dish or light lunch.

13. Fermented Mushroom and Spinach Omelette

Prep Time: 10 minutes
Cook Time: 10 minutes
Ingredients:

- 3 large eggs
- 2 tablespoons milk
- 1 cup sliced mushrooms
- 1 cup fresh spinach leaves
- 1/4 cup diced onion
- 1 clove garlic, minced
- 2 tablespoons olive oil
- Salt and pepper to taste

Instructions:

1. In a bowl, whisk together the eggs and milk until well combined. Set aside.

2. Use a non-stick skillet to heat olive oil on medium heat setting.

3. Add diced onion and minced garlic to the skillet. Sauté for 2-3 minutes until fragrant and onions are translucent.

4. Add sliced mushrooms to the skillet and cook for another 3-4 minutes until they start to brown.

5. Add fresh spinach leaves to the skillet and cook for 1-2 minutes until wilted.

6. Season the mushroom and spinach mixture with salt and pepper to taste.

7. Remove the vegetable mixture from the skillet and set aside.

8. Reduce the heat to low and pour the whisked eggs into the skillet.

9. Allow the eggs to cook undisturbed for a minute until the edges start to set.

10. Using a spatula, gently lift the edges of the omelette and tilt the skillet to let the uncooked eggs flow to the edges.

11. Once the eggs are mostly set but still slightly runny on top, spoon the mushroom and spinach mixture onto one half of the omelette.

12. Fold the other half of the omelette over the filling to form a half-moon shape.

13. Cook for an additional 1-2 minutes to ensure the eggs are fully cooked and the filling is heated through.

14. Slide the omelette onto a plate and serve hot as a delicious and protein-packed breakfast or brunch option.

14. Fermented Lentil Soup

Prep Time: 10 minutes

Cook Time: 30 minutes

Ingredients:

- 1 cup dried lentils, rinsed
- 4 cups vegetable broth
- 1 onion, chopped
- 2 carrots, diced
- 2 celery stalks, diced
- 2 cloves garlic, minced
- 2 tablespoons olive oil
- 1 teaspoon ground cumin
- 1 teaspoon paprika
- 1/2 teaspoon turmeric
- Salt and pepper to taste
- 2 tablespoons lemon juice
- Chopped fresh parsley for garnish

Instructions:
1. Use a large pot to heat olive oil on medium heat setting.
2. Add chopped onion, diced carrots, and diced celery. Gently cook the vegetables for a duration of 5 minutes, allowing them to gradually tenderize.
3. Add minced garlic, ground cumin, paprika, turmeric, salt, and pepper. Continue cooking for an extra 1-2 minutes until a delightful aroma fills the air.
4. Place the rinsed lentils into the pot along with the vegetable broth. Bring to a boil.
5. Reduce heat to low, cover the pot, and simmer for 20-25 minutes until the lentils are tender.
6. Stir in lemon juice and adjust the seasoning if needed.
7. Take out of the heat and allow the soup cool down a bit.
8. Using an immersion blender or a countertop blender, puree about half of the soup until smooth. Leave some lentils and vegetables intact for texture.
9. Return the soup to the pot and heat over low heat for a few more minutes to warm it through.
10. Ladle the fermented lentil soup into bowls.
11. Garnish with chopped fresh parsley.
12. Serve the soup hot as a comforting and nutritious meal.

15. Fermented Salmon Salad
Prep Time: 10 minutes
Ingredients:
- 8 ounces cooked salmon, flaked
- 2 cups mixed salad greens
- 1/2 cup cherry tomatoes, halved

- 1/4 cup sliced red onion
- 2 tablespoons capers
- 2 tablespoons extra virgin olive oil
- 1 tablespoon lemon juice
- Salt and pepper to taste

Instructions:
1. In a large bowl, combine the flaked salmon, mixed salad greens, cherry tomatoes, sliced red onion, and capers.
2. In a small bowl, whisk together the extra virgin olive oil, lemon juice, salt, and pepper.
3. Delicately pour the dressing over the salad, gently tossing the mixture to ensure every component is evenly coated.
4. Adjust the seasoning if needed.
5. Transfer the salmon salad to a serving plate or bowl.
6. Enjoy the fermented salmon salad as a light and flavorful meal.

16. Fermented Banana Bread
Prep Time: 15 minutes
Cook Time: 1 hour
Ingredients:
- 3 ripe bananas, mashed
- 1/2 cup sugar
- 1/4 cup melted butter
- 1/4 cup plain yogurt
- 2 eggs
- 1 teaspoon vanilla extract

- 1 1/2 cups all-purpose flour
- 1 teaspoon baking soda
- 1/2 teaspoon salt

Instructions:

1. Preheat the oven to 350°F (175°C). Prepare a loaf pan by applying a thin layer of grease and keep it aside.

2. In a large bowl, combine the mashed bananas, sugar, melted butter, plain yogurt, eggs, and vanilla extract. Mix well.

3. Combine the all-purpose flour, baking soda, and salt in a separate bowl with a whisk.

4. Carefully incorporate the powdered components into the banana blend, gently stirring until fully integrated. Be careful not to overmix.

5. Transfer the batter into the greased loaf pan and use a spatula to ensure the top surface is even and level.

6. Put the batter into the oven that has been preheated and allow it to bake for around 60 minutes or until an inserted toothpick reveals no traces of batter when removed.

7. Remove the banana bread from the oven and let it cool in the pan for 10 minutes.

8. Move the loaf of bread to a wire rack for complete cooling prior to slicing.

9. Slice and serve the fermented banana bread as a delightful and comforting treat.

17. Fermented Kimchi Fried Rice

Prep Time: 10 minutes
Cook Time: 15 minutes
Ingredients:

- 2 cups cooked rice, preferably day-old
- 1 cup kimchi, chopped
- 1/2 cup diced carrots
- 1/2 cup frozen peas
- 2 cloves garlic, minced
- 1 tablespoon vegetable oil
- 1 tablespoon soy sauce
- 1 teaspoon sesame oil
- 2 green onions, chopped
- 2 eggs (optional)
- Salt and pepper to taste

Instructions:
1. Use a large skillet or wok to heat vegetable oil on medium heat setting.
2. Add minced garlic and diced carrots to the skillet. Sauté for 2-3 minutes until the carrots start to soften.
3. Add frozen peas and chopped kimchi to the skillet. Stir-fry for another 2-3 minutes until the kimchi is heated through.
4. Push the vegetables to one side of the skillet and crack the eggs into the empty space. Scramble the eggs until cooked.
5. Add cooked rice to the skillet and stir to combine with the vegetables and eggs.

6. Slowly pour soy sauce and sesame oil onto the rice medley. Toss well to evenly coat.

7. Cook for an additional 3-4 minutes, stirring occasionally, until the fried rice is heated through.

8. Enhance the flavor by adding salt and pepper to your liking.

9. Remove from heat and stir in chopped green onions.

10. Serve the fermented kimchi fried rice hot as a satisfying and flavorful meal.

18. Fermented Pineapple Salsa

Prep Time: 15 minutes

Ingredients:

- 2 cups diced fresh pineapple
- 1/2 cup diced red bell pepper
- 1/4 cup diced red onion
- 1 jalapeno pepper, finely chopped and free of seeds
- 1/4 cup chopped fresh cilantro
- 2 tablespoons lime juice
- 1 tablespoon honey
- Salt to taste

Instructions:

1. In a bowl, combine the diced fresh pineapple, diced red bell pepper, diced red onion, finely diced jalapeno pepper, and chopped cilantro.

2. Use a separate small bowl to whisk together the lime juice and honey.

3. Pour the lime juice and honey mixture over the pineapple salsa ingredients.
4. Toss well to combine and coat the salsa evenly.
5. Season with salt to taste.
6. Let the salsa sit for at least 10 minutes to allow the flavors to meld together.
7. Serve the fermented pineapple salsa as a refreshing and tangy condiment or topping for grilled meats, tacos, or tortilla chips.

19. Fermented Chickpea Salad
Prep Time: 10 minutes
Ingredients:
- 2 cups cooked chickpeas
- 1 cup diced cucumber
- 1/2 cup cherry tomatoes, halved
- 1/4 cup diced red onion
- 1/4 cup chopped fresh parsley
- 2 tablespoons lemon juice
- 2 tablespoons extra virgin olive oil
- Salt and pepper to taste

Instructions:
1. In a large bowl, combine the cooked chickpeas, diced cucumber, cherry tomatoes, diced red onion, and chopped fresh parsley.
2. Combine the lemon juice, extra virgin olive oil, salt, and pepper in a small bowl with a whisk.
3. Pour the dressing over the chickpea salad ingredients.

4. Toss well to coat the salad evenly with the dressing.
5. Adjust the seasoning if needed.
6. Let the chickpea salad sit for a few minutes to allow the flavors to blend.
7. Serve the fermented chickpea salad as a nutritious and protein-packed side dish or light meal.

20. Fermented Chocolate Banana Smoothie

Prep Time: 5 minutes
Ingredients:
- 2 ripe bananas
- 1 cup milk (dairy or plant-based)
- 1/4 cup Greek yogurt
- 2 tablespoons unsweetened cocoa powder
- 1 tablespoon of honey, alternatively, maple syrup (optional for added sweetness)
- 1/2 cup ice cubes

Instructions:
1. Peel the ripe bananas and place them in a blender.
2. Add milk, Greek yogurt, unsweetened cocoa powder, and honey or maple syrup (if using).
3. Add ice cubes to the blender.
4. Blend on high speed until all the ingredients are well combined and the smoothie is creamy and smooth.
5. Taste the smoothie and adjust the sweetness or cocoa powder amount according to your preference.
6. Pour the fermented chocolate banana smoothie into glasses.
7. Serve immediately as a delicious and indulgent treat or a satisfying breakfast-on-the-go.

Conclusion

Embracing an anti-Parkinson diet centered around fermented foods can have a profound impact on managing the symptoms of Parkinson's disease. The journey of John, our protagonist, serves as a testament to the potential benefits of this approach.

Through his research and experimentation, he discovered that improving gut health through the consumption of fermented foods can positively influence brain function and reduce inflammation.

The collection of 20 delicious, quick, and easy-to-make recipes provided in this cookbook offers a diverse range of options to incorporate fermented ingredients into your daily meals. From tangy fermented black bean tacos to comforting lentil soup and refreshing pineapple salsa, each recipe is thoughtfully designed to provide both nourishment and flavor.

By following this anti-Parkinson diet and integrating these recipes into your culinary repertoire, you can embark on a path of enhanced well-being and symptom management. Remember, this cookbook is just the beginning. Explore the realm of fermented foods, experiment with flavors, and adapt the recipes to suit your preferences and dietary needs.

Together, let us continue to explore alternative approaches to managing Parkinson's disease and empower ourselves with knowledge and delicious recipes to promote gut health, reduce inflammation, and ultimately improve our overall quality of life.

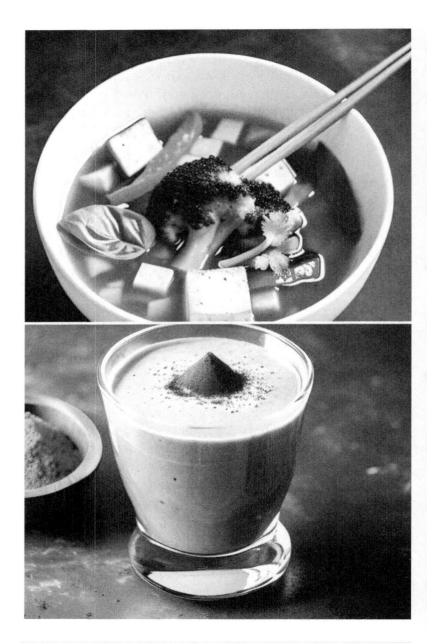

Printed in Great Britain
by Amazon

44385615R00020

About the Book

Introducing the "Parkinson's Disease Diet Recipes Cookbook," your
ultimate companion on the journey to managing and reversing
Parkinson's disease. Packed with mouthwatering recipes, this guide
is specifically designed for those newly diagnosed with Parkinson's,
offering a powerful dietary approach to improve their quality of life.

In the comprehensive introduction, you'll gain an understanding of
how nutrition plays a pivotal role in the management of Parkinson's
disease. Unlock the secrets of an anti-Parkinson's diet and learn how
specific foods can help combat symptoms, reduce inflammation, and
support brain health.

Featuring 20 delectable recipes, each carefully crafted with
wholesome ingredients (and include simple step-by-step cooking
instruction and preparation time), this cookbook will inspire you to
embrace a nourishing and flavorful approach to your meals. From
fermented kefir smoothie bowls to tempting kimchi fried rice,
sauerkraut and turkey lettuce wraps to irresistible fermented
chocolate banana smoothies, every recipe is not only delicious but
also designed to provide essential nutrients for your body.

Take control of your health and embark on a culinary journey that
combines taste and well-being. This cookbook is your gateway to a
healthier and happier life, where every meal becomes an opportunity
to thrive.

Don't let Parkinson's disease define you—empower yourself with the
"Parkinson's Disease Diet Recipes Cookbook" today.

Transform your health and reverse the effects of Parkinson's disease
with this dietary book.

Order your copy now and embrace a delicious and nourishing journey
to a better life!

ISBN 9798397856898

9 798397 856898